Ignite Your Creativity and Stoke Your Compassion

40 Essential Yoga Postures

Ignite Your Creativity and Stoke Your Compassion
40 Essential Yoga Postures
2019

FIRST EDITION

Library of Congress Cataloging-in-Publication Data has been applied for.

ISBN: 978-1-704-53917-1 (pbk)

1.Yoga I. Title.

For everyone
who has taught me
how to appreciate what is
create what could be
and laugh at it all.

CONTENTS

Firefly

Tortoise

Fish

Corpse

Preface

This book is intended as a yoga practice companion rather than a yoga practice manual. There are literally thousands of yoga books on what to do and how to do yoga postures. There are literally tens if not hundreds of thousands of yoga teachers who can tell you where to put your foot or how to use a yoga prop. If you show up at a yoga class or workshop that I am teaching, I would be happy to show you the ins and outs of the what and the how of yoga. However, this book is not intended to be used for that purpose. Instead, this is an exploration of the why. This is an inquiry into the what, how, and why to use your mind in a yoga practice.

The reason that who, where and when are not mentioned above is that the who is you, the where is literally anywhere you are, and the when is always right now. You don't need to be someone in particular to be able to practice yoga. You don't need to be anywhere in particular to practice yoga. You don't need to practice at any particular time. These have been and continue to be stumbling blocks for people who use the time, place, and person to discourage themselves from practicing yoga. Here are some of the common excuses people give: "I don't have enough time." "This isn't the right time. I'll do it later." "I don't have the right clothes." "I don't know the names of the postures." "I'm not flexible." "My house is too cluttered." "I have too many things to do." "I've never done yoga before." "I used to do yoga, so I'll do it again when I am in as good a shape as I was then." "I don't know how to do yoga." "I'm too old." "I'm too young." "I'm too muscular." "I'm too weak." "I'm too big." "I'm too sick." "I already workout in other ways." "I'm not spiritual." "I am spiritual." "I tried yoga once and it was too hard."

You might resonate with one or more of these or maybe you have other reasons why you feel like you need to be more or different than you are in order to enjoy practicing yoga, reasons why the place matters, or reasons why the time is not right. If you get nothing else from this book, at least get this:

YOU ARE ENOUGH.

RIGHT WHERE YOU ARE IS THE PERFECT PLACE.

NOW IS THE TIME.

Introduction

Yoga is a practice of being and becoming a more honest, kind, compassionate, caring, considerate, thoughtful, and mindful human being. Often yoga practice has been and is being marketed for its side effects: increased balance, strength, flexibility, bone density, heart health, anxiety and depression reduction, overall reduced health care costs and personal quality of life. While all of this is often true for most people who practice yoga, it is not and has not been the reason for yoga's development and flourishing. In other words, if practicing yoga doesn't seem to make you more honest, kind, compassionate, caring, considerate, thoughtful, and/or mindful someone is either not really teaching you yoga or you are not practicing yoga correctly.

While much has been written about the origins of yoga, we are still left with a great deal of uncertainty about not only its inception, but its continued evolution through the centuries. What we do know is that yoga, like art, music, science, and medicine is a human invention. Despite some human claims to divine inspiration and direct deity intervention, people have been and continue to be responsible for the development of yoga. We would do ourselves and the yoga practice a service by more consistently and boldly acknowledging and celebrating the human creativity that lies at the heart of yoga practice.

This creativity gets squelched by the mythos of and adherence to religious dogma as it relates to yoga practice. The power of the creative mind is further limited by the insistence upon the notions that lineage is sacred and that some past or present human's yogic abilities inherently supersedes our own. An embrace of yoga's creative core need not be a shunning of its history or the contributions of past practitioners. To the contrary, the creative development of yoga in this moment is dependent upon the foundations of practice already laid. But simply tending to the preservation of the foundation does not build the structure. Mindful use of what we already know, a constant questioning of what, how and why we know these things, and a dedication to continued growth and development keep yoga alive and growing.

The primary purpose of yoga practice is to create, strengthen or reveal connection, integration, and union. This is one of the reasons why so many of the yoga postures are named after the natural world. Creators of yoga asana assumed physical positions to develop, enhance, and illuminate mental and emotional connections with the world they saw around them. A superficial understanding of these connections assumes that the postures are meant to mimic what we see in the world: the tree pose looks like a tree, the fish pose looks like a fish, the frog pose looks like a frog, etc. However, some deeper scrutiny reveals that not all of the postures really look like their namesakes. Does the camel really look like a camel? What about the cow face? How about locust? In fact, it is our creative mind that allows us to even make a connection between the names of the postures and what the creatures and structures they are named for really look like. In other words, if you did an experiment where you took people who had never done yoga, or preferably even really seen or heard of it (to be fair, I'm not really sure who those people are at the this point, but the thought experiment still holds) and showed them people doing the positions of yoga postures, my guess is that the likelihood is extremely low that they would name the postures, tree, fish, frog, camel, cow face, locust, and all the rest.

For someone who cares deeply about connection, integration, and union, are the superficialities of the external expression the only things that matter? No. This is not to suggest that the names of the yoga postures are arbitrary. Instead it is that they are named not simply for their external appearance, but rather, primarily for their internal experience. If yoga practice is truly about connecting and integrating then we must engage in contemplating what it must feel like to be a tree, fish, frog, etc. Of course, with the structures of our brains we can never really know what it is like to be some other being. However, in the attempt we open up lines of understanding. Just as we can never really know what it is like to be another human being, but in making attempts at understanding we create stronger bonds of compassion and caring.

Section 1: The Natural World

As we explore those postures named for the world we see around us, let us commit to opening our minds to deeper understanding. Let us use our creativity to imagine not just mimic. Let us feel not just look. Let us listen with open minds and hearts to the union that already exists but is not yet revealed and for the opportunities to create new bonds of connection.

Mountain

"In my mind's eye, I visualize how a particular sight and feeling will appear on a print. It is an intuitive sense and an ability that comes from a lot of practice." – Ansel Adams

What does it feel like to "be" a mountain? How can you embody those qualities of being? Certainly a mountain is massive, grounded, a part of the earth itself. It is also tall, broad, and expands into the sky. We often think of the mountain as stable and unmoving, steadfast and majestic. A mountain is, however, also in motion. At first glance we might miss this motion because it is happening at a geologic pace. With more careful observation the movements of the mountain become more apparent and our ability to embody them more accessible.

As you practice a mountain posture let go of attempting to stop motion. Let go of the idea that your body must reach and then maintain a particular position. Instead, practice moving very, very slowly. Do this in the way that you distribute weight on your feet at the foundation. Instead of shifting your feet rapidly, in order to find what you preconceive of as "the right position" as quickly as possible, slowly make yourself aware of how you are already carrying the weight in your feet. Do the same with your legs, hips, abdomen, back, shoulders, arms, hands, neck, and head.

Continue to consider the way that a mountain changes. Wind blows across its face, moving dust from the mountain's surface. Flora grows from its top soil, slowly growing, by taking up the minerals that make up the mountain itself. Sun heats the surface of rock, melts ice, and warms water. The water from rain, sleet, and snow run through crags and crevices, in rivers, streams, and creeks, causing erosion, changing the very shape of the mountain. How can you embody these subtle changes? Feel your breath like wind or rain changing the experience of being in your body.

Often the mountain changes slightly, but a buildup of these seemingly little changes can result in bigger ones. A small pebble loosened by a tiny animal or the wind can be the final catalyst for a seemingly cataclysmic mudslide, rock slide, or avalanche. Volcanic activity can seem sudden and unexpectedly violent. The earth's molten core has been churning for eons, but what we experience on the outside is that from its depths, the mountain explodes its core and in a sense is reborn as something new and deeply changed. But this change was a long time coming. What has been brewing under your surface, at your depths? Be aware of the small changes that might lead to an avalanche of transformation or an eruption of something essentially you.

Although we cannot see it even in our whole lifetime, we know that the genesis of the mountain is the geologic movement of the very crust of the earth itself, its tectonic plates squeezing into one another, driving the mountains higher and steeper. Consider the foundations of what drives you to grow, the energy that moves you to develop, and the power you have deep within to reach ever higher.

Allow these considerations to inform the way that your feet stand upon the earth, the way that your head moves into the sky, and the way that your body broadens into the space surrounding you. With this reflection upon what it is like to be a mountain find a deeper patience, a willingness to take a longer view of your actions, less urgency to get to a final

form, and an understanding of the constant flow of change
of which you are a part.

Dog

"Yesterday I was a dog. Today I'm a dog. Tomorrow I'll
probably still be a dog. There's so little hope for
advancement."
– Snoopy (From "Peanuts" By Charles Shultz)

Think about a dog taking a nap: curled up and content.
Then imagine the dog waking up from its slumber. Often
the first thing that the dog does is stretch out its front legs
and then its back legs. The dog does this first because it
feels good, like when you wake up from a nap it feels good
to stand and stretch your arms to the sky. Another reason
the dog does this is that it gets the blood flowing and allows
for a full open breath. Stretching out the legs in these ways
gets the dog ready for moving, for walking, or even
running.

Now imagine that you are that dog. All of your basic daily
needs are taken care of by someone else, someone that you
trust and who trusts you. When you awaken from a nap or
even first thing in the morning you feel a general sense of
safety and this gives you a feeling of freedom. When you
move into the downward or upward facing dog postures
embody this feeling of preparing for broader movement in
the context of feeling safe and secure.

In the downward dog, feel free to wag your tail a little as
you stretch out your arms, legs, shoulders, and hips.
Imagine the possibilities of movement that could flow from
this new found space in your body. In the upward dog, feel
free to smile, stretching out your face as you open your
chest and shoulders. Good dog.

Cobra

"Ride the snake. Ride the snake, to the lake, the ancient lake baby." – The Doors

You are a cobra. You have no arms or legs. Your whole body is a powerful coil of muscles. Your movements are smooth and controlled. While you mostly move along the earth, your strength has the power to lift most of your body up from the ground to face potential danger, to enjoy potential sustenance, and to simply experience the feeling of uplift. When your body does rise from the earth, you create a base of coiled support, a store of energy like a spring, that propels you upward and outward. In this position your forward and upward movement is lead from your chest, not your head. When potential danger has passed, or you have taken in what is needed, and you are ready to move on or rest, then you ease your way back down to the earth calmly and carry on quietly.

Cat

"Cats are connoisseurs of comfort." – James Herriot

Cats are a collection of contradictions, alternately calm and aggressive, graceful and abrupt, affectionate and distant. When we take on the actions of the cat in yoga we embrace not only the physicality of the cat, but these internal contradictions as well. The pompous puss lifts both its head and tail simultaneously while the frightened feline buries both its top and bottom for protection. Alternate between these two positions, breath by breath. What does it feel like to be completely open in one moment and then in the next moment as closed as can be? Explore the vacillation between courage and cowardice. You, like all of us, can be both deeply afraid and deeply bold at the same time. You can make yourself vulnerable while maintaining an inner protection.

Pigeon

"I like pigeons." – Bert from Sesame Street

A lot of the language used in yoga classes, books, videos, and even conversation involves the notion of yoga being a way to elevate oneself, to find your best self, to grow, develop, and become more, even better. In many ways, this is certainly true. However, what some people miss is that elevation in the yogic sense is about enhanced recognition of or experience of connection. This expanding understanding of integration must include not only those beings we often deem powerful, majestic, and awe-inspiring, but also those creatures that are usually derided, dirty, and downtrodden. Few beings embody this as well as the pigeon.

As you practice the pigeon you find yourself quite close to the ground. In the downward facing/forward bending variation that is commonly practiced your face is in fact on the ground. The energy of this variation is one of dropping deeper and deeper downward toward the earth, not just with your face, but with your whole body: legs, hips, chest, arms, and head. How can you find ease in this descent?

Then there is the upward facing/backward bending variation, from which the posture derives its name. While the pigeon is oft considered nothing more than "a flying rat", when it stands and walks, it does so with head and heart held high. While it is often associated with the dirtiest parts of our world, it still has the ability to alight and to soar. Can you find the ability to be at peace with your lowest self while also lifting up to your highest? As you become the pigeon, let go into the earth and lighten into the sky.

Tree

"I kick it root down. I put my root down. I kick it
down. I put my root down. So how we gonna kick it?
Gonna kick it root down. So how you wanna kick it?
Gonna kick it root down. So how you gonna kick it? Gonna
kick it root down. Gonna break it on down. Gonna kick it
root down." – Beastie Boys

Stop what you are doing and look outside. If you're already outside, look around. Once you see a tree, look at it closely, deeply. It doesn't matter what kind of tree it is or if you can identify its variety. As you look at the tree think about its lifespan and where it might be in that span. Is it very young, very old, middle aged? How can you tell? Where is its parent? What was its life like? What about the generation before that? And before that? Once you've considered the long lineage of this tree, now consider its potential progeny. Will it bear young? Where and how will they live? What about their offspring?

Now return your awareness to this tree as it is right now. There are clearly things about this tree that you can see. Does it currently have leaves? Did it have leaves at some point? Will it have leaves again in the future? How tall and wide is its trunk? What is the texture of its bark? How prolific are its branches? What are all the parts of the tree that you can see? Now consider all the parts of the tree that you cannot see, but can imagine. Whatever size the tree is above ground think about how intricate and powerful the roots of this tree must be below ground in order to provide a foundation of stability and balance. Think about the myriad processes going on right now within the tree to convert sunlight into energy and to draw nutrients and water from the earth. While the tree cannot speak, you can surely listen. What do you hear?

As you practice the tree posture consider the ways in which you might embody what you observe in the tree. Start from the foundation. One mistake yoga practitioners make in the tree posture is that they imagine that the roots of the tree are just that, imaginary. I've heard many a yoga teacher suggest that students, "Imagine roots reaching down through the sole of your foot and into the earth, grounding your posture…" or something along those lines. When you practice a yoga posture, don't just make parts of the posture imaginary extensions of your body, actual make every part of your body a part of the posture. So instead of creating imaginary roots, simply re-imagine where the ground begins. Look at the tree again. Is the base of the trunk wider or narrower than the top of the trunk? Wider. So, if the trunk of your body is the trunk of the tree, then your legs are not a strangely narrow portion of the trunk that happens to be even taller than the rest of the trunk. No. Your legs are the roots of the tree. The ground level is at your hips and/or waist, your trunk is the trunk, and your arms, hands, fingers, neck, and head are the branches and potentially leaves. When you conceptualize the ground at your hips it can create a stronger feeling of stability coming from your center. When you feel the legs as roots, instead of trying to hold them rigidly like a trunk, you free them to open and move and stretch out into the earth surrounding them. When your legs and trunk are experienced this way, then you will feel more confident in stretching out branches into the space surrounding you. When you come out of the tree posture, move your lifted leg like a root reaching deeper into the earth.

Eagle

"Eagles come in all shapes and sizes, but you will
recognize them chiefly by their attitudes."
– E.F. Schumacher

Most of us do not have regular contact with eagles as
frequently as we do with beings like dogs, cats, trees, and
pigeons. Our frame of reference therefore with regard to
eagles is often less personal and more socially or culturally
filtered. Take a moment to let your filters with regard to
eagles fall away. Let go of the idea that you are looking at
eagles and trying to be like what you have seen. Instead,
once again, engage your creative mind. What must it be
like to nest so high? How about to soar? What about the
speed with which you swoop down upon your prey? Prior
to and following the swoop how does it feel to perch, to sit
patiently, to preen, to peer out the world stretched out in
front of you?

As you begin your practice of eagle, start from that place of
safety and stability in your perch. Instead of thinking that
you are attempting to cross your arms as tightly as possible,
turn your attention to the back of your body and focus on
spreading your wings (shoulder blades) broadly. As your
legs cross over each other, focus on the feeling of soaring,
not an insecure attempt at standing on one leg. Engage your
legs and arms as if you were swooping down from high in
the sky and let the pull of gravity draw you down toward
the earth. Then smoothly return to your perch, to sit
patiently, to preen, and to peer out at the world stretched
out in front of you.

Moon

Yoga is a long term practice. Sure it might feel good in the moment to stretch a hip or a shoulder, and yes, you will likely feel better having engaged in a single practice session. Certainly there is power in a moment of awareness, a moment of freedom. However, the depth of unity embodied in the yoga practice is best experienced and strengthened by consistent practice, over and over again. So it is with our experience of the moon. Certainly, we may be awed by its beauty in a given moment, whether it is full, half, quarter, or crescent. But our deeper understanding of the moon and our sincere appreciation of its beauty, its presence, and its power comes from repeated, consistent observation.

Our perception of the moon is in constant flux because of the relationship between sun, earth, and moon. It is not that the moon itself waxes and wanes; it is our perception that is waxed and waned by the light of the sun reflected to us by the moon. In other words, the whole moon is always "there"; however, our ability to see the moon is dependent upon where we are in the lunar cycle. This awareness has relevance in our practice of the half moon posture. As you stand upon one leg the other is lifted behind you and out of sight. Your ability to see either arm will depend upon whether you choose to look down towards the ground, out to the horizon, or up to the sky. In truth, the half moon posture is more like a crescent moon in terms of how much of your body you actually see (i.e. very little). However, your lack of external vision in no way limits your internal awareness of your body. Without looking at your lifted foot, flex it at the ankle and press out through the foot like you are standing on it. Without looking at your standing leg, unlock your knee and engage the musculature of your thigh. Without seeing your bottom arm shoulder, release it, and find space between your shoulder and your neck.

The moon is not only an object to be seen it is also a subject that acts upon the earth. In a way that cannot be seen, but can still be understood, the moon, some 238,900 miles from earth, commands the tides of our oceans. Likewise, although we cannot see it, our very breath commands the tides of our lives. While practicing any of the moon postures deeply consider the tide of your breath, the rise and fall upon the ocean of your body. Watch the way that even without any physical effort on your part, your body expands and opens up with each inhalation and contracts and falls away with each exhalation. As you engage your body in the actions of the posture, allow this invisible pull of breath to move you into broader opening and deeper softening.

Crane

"I will write peace on your wings and you will fly all over
the world." - Sadako Sasaki

While as human beings we might imagine that the Crane
posture resembles flight, upon careful consideration we are
compelled to acknowledge that while we are the closest we
might come to alighting, we are still firmly on the ground.
What is also apparent is that we are standing no longer
upon the power, strength, and volume of our legs, but upon
the shaky foundation of our arms. And yet, our arms are
broader still than the legs of the crane. So then how does it
stand so firmly in the flow of a river or the unstable soil of
the river's banks with legs so thin and spindly? How does it
not only find balance, but look about, and even find
sustenance upon those legs? More importantly how do you
emulate that ability as you practice the crane?

The best way is to embrace the idea of grounding is to build
a foundation and release the notion that you must fly in
order to succeed. Spread your fingers broadly upon the
ground and grip the earth firmly with your fingers, like the
crane burying its feet in the mud. Instead of trying to lift up
at first, press down with your arms and hands. Your
shoulder blades are your wings. Let them spread wide and
let your back round. Tuck your legs in deeply to your trunk
and your arms, for what once were your arms, are now your
legs. And once grounded firmly, when you move to lift up
toward the sky, do it from the highest points of your body
first, likely your hips, lower abdomen, and what once were
your legs, but are now a tail of plumage.

It is important to note here that the crane posture described
above is sometimes also called crow. While technically

these are really two different postures, in practice they often look the same. This appearance of similarity is confounded by the way that crane and crow sound and are therefore transliterated into English as bakasana and kakasana respectively. You might try saying bakasana and kakasana out loud and notice how similar they sound. Then imagine that a native English speaker is attempting to discern the difference by listening to a non-native English speaker and you can quickly perceive how this confusion arose quite easily.

As a reminder, for our purposes, these distinctions are essentially irrelevant. What is relevant is what you imagine it might feel like to be a crane. Then imagine what it might feel like to be a crow. It is readily apparent that when taking on the feeling of being a crow, your legs are much shorter and therefore your body and center of gravity are much closer to the ground. The crow is much more hunkered down and compact, while the crane is almost flamboyant in its height and litheness. While both yoga postures require placing all of your body weight onto your arms and hands, in one, that weight is lightened to the sky and in the other, that weight is born to sink deeper into the earth. Enjoy the experience of alternating between these contrasting experiences of being: crane and crow.

Cow

"Don't have a cow man." – Bart Simpson

Few postures inspire queries regarding the correlation
between posture name and the way a posture looks as
Gomukasana, the cow face pose. While the inquiry is
welcome, again, this particular question misses the essence
of the practice. We are less concerned with looking like a
cow's face and more concerned with feeling like a cow or
more specifically the face of a cow. Cows display a kind of
serenity. Even when chewing, which they are often doing,
the chew is slow and methodical, contented and relaxed. So
as you take the actions of the posture, slowly and
methodically cross your legs one over the other. Be relaxed
and content as one arm goes behind and gradually up your
back and the other goes up and over behind your neck.
Practice the posture as if you had nothing else but this to do
all day (even though you may have many things to do). Let
go of your attachment to achieving hands that touch behind
your back and be content to practice opening your heart,
your hips, your shoulders, and your mind.

Camel

"Are you in a desert? Then be a camel! Be compatible with the reality." – Mehmet Murat ildan

How far are you prepared to travel? Like a camel carrying a heavy load, what burdens have you been carrying? The camel travels long distances slowly, rather than short distances quickly. You are in this for the long haul. Take your time packing and preparing for your journey. Set your foundation mindfully. Build strength purposefully in your legs: press down into the earth with your shins, squeeze your inner thighs inward, and pull your front thighs upward. Stabilize your lower back with the strength of your lower abdomen. Engage the strength of your neck by drawing your chin downward to start. Know that your journey as a camel will require a long term commitment to these actions, that you must, regardless of how tired you become, carry on. Then as you continue to engage these foundational actions, very slowly, with no urgency, lift your heart to the sky. Even though you are weighed down with heavy burdens, you have the capacity to endure. Notice the length of the back of your neck and maintain as much of that space as you can, while you open your throat and front of your neck gradually. Your hands may best be used for support on your back, at your hips, or on your feet, but do not be overly distracted by how far your hands are able to reach. Instead continue to look up and out at the vast journey ahead.

Frog

"When green is all there is to be, it could make you wonder
why. But why wonder why?"
– Kermit The Frog
(From "Rainbow Connection" By Paul Williams and
Kenneth Ascher)

Consider the amphibious nature of frogs. They are
adaptable, able to survive in or out of the water. Practice
embodying that adaptability as you kneel down, sit back
toward your haunches, move your legs away from each
other and stretch your trunk, arms, and head out in front of
you. You may choose to keep your feet together as your
legs move wide or you may choose to move your feet apart
from each other at the same width as your knees. You may
choose to continue sitting back with your hips toward your
heels or you may move your hips forward as far as the
invisible line that runs from knee to knee. Wherever you
practice, continue to be adaptable. Be open to change as it
unfolds. Be ready to shift position to accommodate a
shifting environment. Feel free to play with bringing your
head and trunk down into the depths of the posture, like the
frog in the water. But also experiment with keeping your
head and trunk up out of the depths. Neither is better than
the other. Each is simply a different environment in which
you can explore being. O.K., hop to it.

Locust

"You have great powers, only some of which you have as
yet discovered."
– Jor-El to his son Kal-El
(From "Superman" By Jerry Siegel)

It is one thing to commune with, to attempt to empathize
with, or to emulate creatures that are often of service to
human beings or at least cause us little to no harm, but to
practice "being" creatures who are perceived to cause us
harm is truly at the core of what it means to engage in an
intentional practice of yoga, truly connecting and
understanding. So as you envision becoming a locust,
embody the desire of all living creatures to simply survive.
Engage in compassion as much as any muscular action.

Locusts don't just fly; they fly with precision and focus.
From lying down on your belly, take flight by precisely
activating your legs inward and backward while mobilizing
your trunk to move forward. Create the flight from as close
to your center of gravity as possible so that your arms are
free to soar like wings and your head and neck are free to
observe, identify, and approach the sustenance that drives
you. In other words, relax your neck, fly from your center,
support from your limbs and enjoy the view.

Rabbit

"'Well', said Rabbit, after a long silence in which nobody
thanked him for the nice walk they were having, 'we'd
better get on, I suppose. Which way shall we try?'"
– A.A. Milne

Floppy ears, a twitchy nose, furry and cute, are the ways we
often see rabbits from the outside. But what must it feel like
to be a rabbit on the inside. Find that your power to move
with strength comes from your legs. Press down firmly into
the earth through your big broad feet (formed by the full
length of your lower legs from your knees down to your
toes). Lighten the weight (out of your head and neck) by
lifting (your hips) towards the sky. Use your ears (formed
by your arms) to sense the world around you, to balance
yourself in space.

Imagine burrowing into a deep safe hole. Notice how
protected you feel. Embody this feeling of protection in
your practice of being a rabbit. To be so small and
vulnerable in a treacherous world requires some safe space
engineering ingenuity. By practicing the rabbit posture you
are practicing feeling safe in a world full of real and
imagined dangers. You are hotwiring your nervous
system's need to feel secure by moving into stillness rather
than trying to hop away. Literally turn inward and face
yourself. Be with yourself in your burrow of fortification.
Breathe slowly. Breathe deeply. It's ok. You're ok.

Scorpion

"O conscience, upright and stainless, how bitter a sting to thee is a little fault." – Dante Alighieri

You are fierce. You are powerful. But you don't need to show it off all the time by strutting and crowing. You can keep your powerful venom to yourself until you really need it. As you store up your energy its potential for striking is coiled deep within you. Your strike can be quick and carefully applied.

Slowly build the strength of your upper body. Quietly coil energy into your core. Lift your head, even with your arms planted firmly so that you can see the world in front of you. Join your legs together to form a powerful tail. There is no need to force your feet, which have become a sharply pointed stinger, over your head, but be ready at any moment to see where you are striking and move the tail and stinger with precision and power.

Lotus

"Everyone knows we need to have mud for lotuses to grow. The mud doesn't smell so good, but the lotus flower smells very good. If you don't have mud, the lotus won't manifest. You can't grow lotus flowers on marble. Without mud, there can be no lotus." – Thich Nhat Hanh

When we ask ourselves what if feels like to be another being we are often tempted not to deeply understand the perspective of this being, but instead to anthropomorphize the being and simply make it conform to our human perspective. This is particularly hazardous as we attempt to better understand beings who we perceive to be less like ourselves, like plants.

In order to imagine that you are a lotus, you must first dispense with the way that we perceive the lotus from the outside. Instead of seeing the lotus from the top down, feel it from the inside out. Feel the rooting in muddy water as a kind of foundational fluidity. As you soften the rigidity of your base, grow, spread, and blossom upward and outward.

We give yoga postures names like "lotus" and "half lotus", implying that there can be such a thing as a half of a lotus. In the same way that a human who is missing a limb is not a partial person, but a whole being, a lotus is a lotus by internal genetics not external representation. There is no half lotus posture juxtaposed to a full lotus posture for our purposes. There is only your expression, from the inside, of a lotus. So, regardless of how much the flexibility and strength of your ankles, knees, thighs, hips, and groin allow you to fold your legs, your lotus blooms.

Lion

"I still believe that one day mankind will bow before the altars of God and be crowned triumphant over war and bloodshed, and nonviolent redemptive goodwill proclaimed the rule of the land. And the lion and the lamb shall lie down together and every man shall sit under his own vine and fig tree and none shall be afraid." – Dr. Martin Luther King Jr.

Be quiet. Be powerful. Find your strength in the quiet. Find calm in your power. Without a natural predator you are relatively safe and secure. From this den of safety and security find the freedom to fully express yourself. Shake out your mane. Loosen your jaw. Let the world and all the other creatures in it hear your roar. Experience the volume of that roar backed up by the strength and fluidity of your muscles. Muscles ready to react at a moment's notice to the playful wrestling of a friendly member of your pride or the potential presence of prey. In yoga, your prey is not a prancing gazelle or zebra stopping at the watering hole. Instead, you patiently stalk your truest self. Move methodically in pursuit of this goal, so as not to scare it away overzealously. Patiently wait, with all of your attention focused, for your moment, this moment, to bring the whole power of your being to bear.

Harness the power of your legs by bringing them in, together toward a strong foundation. Unleash the energy of your heart as you stretch it forward and upward. Stretch out the majesty of your arms and neck. Loosen and open your jaw and your throat to access the energy stored within and utilize more fully the energy of breath.

Peacock

"It dances today, my heart, like a peacock it dances, it
dances. It sports a mosaic of passions like a peacock's tail.
It soars to delight, it quests, oh wildly, it dances today, my
heart, like a peacock it dances." – Rabindranath Tagore

If you pay attention you might notice that false modesty
and boastful arrogance are two sides of the same coin of
egoic insecurity. The choice to belittle your beauty, to
downplay your dynamism, to petrify your power, is often
born of insecurity. A healthy respect for the challenge of
the moment is just that, healthy. But when you shrink from
these challenges without giving the full measure of your
being to overcoming, you shrink yourself.

The set of things of which you are incapable is effectively
infinite with comparison to the set of things which you are
able to do. This should not be born as a burden, but rather
is meant to liberate you from needing to dwell on the
impossible. In yoga we are not concerned with what you
cannot do, we are only interested in what you can do.

So be bold. Be brave. Be the best you that you can be. The
beauty of your plumage is only enhanced when you do this.
Lay your forearms upon the ground, as a peacock; these are
your sturdy feet. Press into the earth and, at the same time,
lift your shoulders towards the sky. Allow your hips to
follow the upward movement. Whether both of your feet
stay on the ground, or one of your legs is lifted to the sky,
or both of your legs and feet stretch themselves upward, be
proud of your strength, your resolve, your ability to
lengthen and lift and grow. Just as no two peacocks'
plumages are exactly alike, no two people express their

beauty in exactly the same way. Rejoice in this diversity. Celebrate your beauty.

Heron

"Poise means holding fast to your principles and beliefs
and acting in accordance with them regardless of how bad
or good the situation may be. Know who you are and be
true to yourself." – John Wooden

Taking on the experience of another being is inherently
fraught with challenges. One of those challenges is feeling
awkward. Many times during yoga practice we are
purposely placing ourselves in awkward positions and then
encouraging ourselves to be calm, to be at ease, to simply
be in the awkwardness. Often, whether outside of or within
a yoga practice, when we feel awkward we make attempts
to alleviate that feeling. A deepening yoga practice is not
necessarily one where the outer awkwardness is dissipated,
but rather, depth in yoga flows from acceptance of this
feeling.

As you take on the feeling of being a heron you take on the
awkwardness of both a very long neck and very long and
skinny legs. The imbalanced hip position created by the
different actions of your two legs is not something you
eliminate, it is something to embrace and relax into. The
strangeness of lifting a foot toward your face is not to be
overcome it is to be developed. As you take on the
awkwardness of the heron feel free to reflect upon your
own awkwardness, embrace it, own it, be it.

Firefly

"Lords of spirit, Lords of breath, Lords of fireflies, stars,
and light, Who will keep the world from death? Who will
stop the coming night?" – Madeleine L'Engle

Imagine being bioluminescent. That means you can light
yourself up without burning yourself out. You have the
power to shine. Use that power without fear. Find that the
way that you shine sends a message to the world around
you about who you are. What kind of signals do you want
to deliver? Who are the intended recipients of this
communication? Why does the way that you are in the
world with relationship to others matter to you?

In order to shine its light, the firefly must create just the
right combination of chemicals. The most important of
these is oxygen. Without oxygen the light has no fuel to
burn. Make breath the central focus of your practice. Use
breath to oxygenate your hands and arms as they become
your foundation. Use breath to power the lift of your hips
into the air. Find in breath the energy that opens your legs
outward from each other and also squeezes them inward
toward your arms. Breathe into flight. Breathe into light.
Breathe into landing and find that even when your hips and
legs return to the earth and your arms no longer hold you
up, the light, your light continues to shine bright.

Tortoise

"'Why did you call him tortoise if he wasn't one?' Alice asked. 'We called him tortoise because he taught us,' said the mock turtle…" – Lewis Carroll

Slow down. Way down. Take your time. There is no rush. Focus in this moment and watch the way that the moment itself arises and then falls away. Do that again and again. Watch the way your breath arises and then falls away, again and again. Notice that if you purposely slow down your breathing it gets a little easier to observe each moment of the breath's unfolding. And when this happens, you might notice the little pauses between breaths, as one breath falls away and another begins. You can do this with your thoughts as well. Watch the way that thoughts arise and fall away. When does one thought end and the next begin? Follow a thought back to its origin. Stay with a thought all the way to its disillusion. Take your time. There is no rush. Slow down.

Apply observation to the actions of your body. Slow your actions down in order to make it easier and easier to watch each movement arise and fall away. Imagine that you have hundreds of years to live. With that awareness let the motion of your legs take shape, gradually descend your trunk between your thighs, slowly bring your legs up over your arms and shoulders and lengthen your legs as you do. Your back and hamstrings will be more inclined to cooperate if they are asked to slowly soften into the depth of the bend. Rest in that depth. Be at ease in this moment and in the impermanence of its existence. Relax into the next arising sensation in your body, wave of your breath, thought in your consciousness. There is no rush. Take your time. Slow down. Way down.

Fish

"The water doesn't know how old you are." – Dara Torres

You, like us all, are born of the sea. Deep in your being that ancestry calls to you. Primordial genetics play themselves out in your current form. And here in this moment the sea still exists within you. You are mostly water after all. Somewhere between the first emergence of life in the waters of Earth and this moment, all these many years later, your ancestors were fish in that sea. They swam and dove and ate and spawned and breathed in the fluidity of that existence.

Be as they were and your present day cousins, still of the sea, continue to be. Stretch out your legs like a tail and move through the air and upon the earth like the tail of a fish in water. Open your heart, arch your back, and dip your head back gracefully. Use your peripheral vision to broaden your perspective. Move like you are weightless, buoyant, and free. In this medium there is no up and down defined by the pull of gravity. Is your head upside down or right side up? Perspective is gained not by searching for the horizon, but instead by gauging light and dark, warmth and cold. Decide how to proceed using these parameters. Do not be afraid to explore the darkness and delve into the depths of colder waters, but go there mindfully, always knowing that at any moment of your choosing you can return to warmer waters, bathed in light, like the waters where life first emerged.

"Contemplating the brevity of life brings some perspective to how we use our attention. None of us knows how much time we have in this life. This is your life. The only one you've got. Why not relax and enjoy your life? Really relax, even in the midst of struggle. Even while doing hard work. Even in uncertainty. You don't know how much time you have left. Whatever you do, however seemingly ordinary, you can feel the preciousness of life. And an awareness of death is the doorway into that way of being in the world." – Sam Harris

Many people spend a lot of mental time and energy preparing for what might, could, or should happen in the future. Sometimes this preparation pays off, when the event unfolds favorably. Sometimes events unfold in ways we could not imagine and this use of our mental energy is wasted. However, there is one thing that we all know for sure will be happening to us, yet very few people spend much if any time preparing for it or more importantly, living with the reality of its inevitability. That is, we all will die. Perhaps it's the inevitability that makes the concept seem trite to some. For others fear prevents an honest exploration of demise. Whatever the reason for a lack of attention to the matter of our death, yoga provides us with an opportunity to explore it first hand, in a sense, to practice dying.

Lying down in savasana is certainly an exercise in relaxation. There are some real physical and physiological benefits to the relaxation element of savasana. However, if what we are after is a broader perspective of being, magnified by our experience of the natural world, then savasana offers us even greater opportunities for understanding and compassion. Intentionally recognize that like all other living beings, you will die. If nothing else, you have this one thing in common with all living beings. If you were a dog, cobra, cat, pigeon, tree, eagle, crane, cow, camel, frog, locust, rabbit, scorpion, lotus, lion, peacock, heron, firefly, tortoise, or fish, you would also inevitably die.

So how does this awareness change not simply what you do, but how you do it, the way in which you engage with the world? Acknowledging that you will die can sharpen your appreciation for what it is like to live, as the being that you are, in this world as it is, right now.

Section 2: Human Ingenuity and Creativity

In a sense, yoga is a celebration of human ingenuity itself. While many of its forms are inspired by the natural world, in yoga the inspiration is merely a starting point. Creativity is what allows us to imagine what it might be like to be a different animal, a plant, or even something inanimate like a mountain. It is this same spark of creativity that has driven human beings to utilize the resources of the natural world in new and productive ways, to harness the energy of nature, and to develop tools that leverage this energy. And so, yoga postures celebrate not only what already exists in nature, but also what exists because of human ingenuity.

Fire Log

"For the correct analogy for the mind is not a vessel that
needs filling, but wood that needs igniting." - Plutarch

Strictly speaking, human beings did not "invent" fire. Nor
did we "discover" fire. Fire is as much a part of the natural
world as ice. However, human beings have developed the
ability to *harness and utilize intentionally* the power of fire
which has led to our ability to identify and access the
potential energy stored in not just wood, but other sources
as well. While today we have the power of flight, we can
communicate across the globe at the speed of light, we can
literally move mountains, none of this or most of the other
technological accomplishments of human beings would be
possible without the first crucial step of being able to create
and utilize the light and heat of fire.

In the fire log posture we celebrate this first giant step of
our ancestors by turning the light and heat of that fire
inward. Your legs take the shape of logs stacked either one
on top of or one in front of the other and your trunk rises
like flame from that foundation. The potential energy of the
logs is burned in order to create the release of heat and light
up through your trunk and head. Should you want to feel
the intensity of that heat or better utilize this light, you
might lean your trunk and head forward, closer to the fire.
But beware not to get to close, lest you get burned.

Utilize the light and heat of the fire to better illuminate the
nature of your existence. Like the logs of the fire, you have
enormous potential energy. How will you release that
energy? How will you control that release? How can the
energy of your life best be utilized? These are the questions

to consider as you sit, staring into the fire of your own being.

Boat

"I am sailing into the wind and the dark. But I am doing my best to keep my boat steady and my sails full." – Arthur Ashe

You must build your boat before you can sail it. From a seated position plant your feet on the floor in front of you with your knees bent and place your arms back behind you to support your back. Engage the strength of your inner thighs, pelvic floor, lower abdomen, and muscles that run up the length of your spine. But a good boat need not only be strong and sturdy, it must also be flexible enough not to be broken by the tides it encounters upon the sea. So also soften your jaw, relax your shoulders and find ease surrounding the core of strength. Feel free to stay at the dock where you built your boat for as long as you like. Sometimes it is nice to simply sit on your boat, tethered to the relative security of the dock (your feet planted) and watch the tides rise and fall and the other ships occasionally go by.

When you are feeling ready to set sail, keep your oars in the water (your hands on the floor behind you) and move the bow of your ship (your feet) into the fluidity of the sea (the air). Move slowly at first by keeping your knees bent. When you get your sea legs, then lengthen your legs longer and higher out in front of you. Once you are sailing smoothly, then pull your oars up out of the water as you stretch your arms out in front. Like a ship on the sea, allow yourself to move with the waves of your breath while keeping your course steady and true.

Plank

"Strength does not come from physical capacity. It comes
from an indomitable will." - Mohandas Gandhi

Consider the versatility of a plank. Alone it can be used as
a ramp, a lever, a bridge, a bench, a shelf, a table, and
more. Combined with other planks a single plank expands
its capabilities to become a roof, a floor, a boat, a house, all
kinds of furniture, and more. Imagine the creativity it took
for someone to conceptualize cutting a felled tree into
smooth, uniform, solid pieces that could be used for far
more intricate building than the tree from which they came.
Bring this degree of versatility and imagination to your
practice of plank.

While you certainly want to make yourself strong like a
plank, you also want to maintain a degree of flexibility that
allows for changing circumstances. If working on your
palms and fingers proves problematic for your wrists or
elbows then be flexible in your approach to the plank and
come down to your forearms. Even if your wrists and
elbows are not an issue for you, feel free to try the plank on
your forearms anyway.

Regardless of the hand and arm position, make sure you are
not just doing an upper body strengthening postures, but
instead, you are also intentionally drawing on the strength
of your lower body. Draw your inner thighs inward, lift
your front thighs upward, and engage the muscles of your
pelvic floor and lower abdomen in particular. Broaden the
space between your shoulder blades to activate the muscles
of your side body (seratus). In other words, you can
certainly think of yourself as a single plank with all of its
strength and capacity. But you can also conceive of

yourself as a collection of planks which are significantly stronger and more versatile together than they are alone. Your strength is drawn from your unique singularity and also from your connection to a collective whole.

Warrior

"Courage is the most important of all virtues, because
without courage you cannot practice any other virtue
consistently." – Maya Angelou

People are sometimes confused about the presence of
"Warrior" postures in the lexicon of yoga practice. The
confusion stems from the seeming dissonance of the
connotation of a warrior as war-like in the context of a
practice that purports to promote peace. There are
numerous examples of people who have been the most
courageous champions of non-violence and peace who also
considered themselves and were considered by others to be
warriors: Martin Luther King Jr., Mohandas Gandhi,
Mother Theresa, Thich Nat Hanh, and more. In this context
the term warrior applies to their courage and determination
in the face of seemingly insurmountable opposition to their
causes. It is this concept of the warrior that most relates to
our practice of connecting and reducing suffering. These
are not goals from which we shrink at the first sign of
resistance, but rather engage like warriors and press on
regardless of the degree or intensity of challenges we face.

In the same way that a warrior needs to be adaptable to
changing circumstances, you can engage in multiple
postures of the body which claim the title Warrior. Whether
standing upon one or both feet remain stable, grounded,
and sure footed. Whether facing the challenges of the
moment directly in front of you or from your flank, do not
be afraid to open your heart. Proactively proceed with
courage rather than defensively waiting in fear. Find a
strong center of balance, a place from which you will not
be moved. From this steady core of your being expand

outward into the world. Stretch out your arms wide into the space around you or expansively to the sky. To be clear, courage does not mean blindly following instructions without regard to the consequences. There is nothing courageous, for example, about feeling that you are engaged in an injurious action, but continuing with the action nonetheless. In fact, courage is quite the opposite. Confront the actual circumstance that you face. Make changes to your actions regardless of the expediency, politics, or vanity they expose. What makes you a warrior is the inner core of your strength expressed into the world around you.

Chair

"There must be those among whom we can sit down and
weep and still be counted as warriors. (I make up this
strange, angry packet for you, threaded with love.) I think
you thought there was no such place for you, and perhaps
there was none then, and perhaps there is none now; but we
will have to make it, we who want an end to suffering, who
want to change the laws of history, if we are not to give
ourselves away." – Adrienne Rich

The most important thing about a chair is its dependability.
No one wants to sit down into a chair only to seconds later
find themselves on the floor because the chair was broken.
Therefore, the first thing you want to develop in your
practice of chair is to engage in actions to which you can
commit for the duration of your chair practice. Sometimes
you won't know what these actions are until you try; so
some trial and error may be required to shape the most
dependable chair possible.

Another important feature of chairs is that they allow us to
sit at a table or desk that is elevated from the ground. We
often come into a chair from a straight up standing position,
but the chair itself keeps us from collapsing to the ground.
Create a focus on that uplifted feeling, rather than the
feeling of dropping down. Make your chair posture lighter
and lighter by utilizing the strength of your inner thighs,
core muscles, and the muscles that run up the length of
your spine. Feel free to imagine that you are at a desk or
table to work on something meaningful to you. Perhaps this
meaningful thing comes from your occupation, or maybe
it's a fun project or something creative you've been
meaning to do. In any case, notice that the focus on the

purpose alleviates, if only for a moment, the feeling of having to work to keep your chair lifted.

While chairs are certainly practical, they are also a furnishing that is part of décor. What kind of chair are you exactly? A lazy-boy recliner? An Eames? A dining chair? A desk chair? Are you made of wood? Metal? Plastic? Are you upholstered or raw? How do you want to be perceived? As merely practical, merely decorative, or some combination and to what degree of each? Your answers to these kinds of questions will determine the nuance of your chair posture practice: how much knee bend, how much hip bend, and the position of your arms.

Finally, remember that while a chair seems to be quite solid in its current form it, like everything, is in a state of change. It was not always a chair; it needed to be crafted, molded, built into this shape from whatever natural resource it is constructed. It will not always be a chair; one day it will break and eventually completely disintegrate back into the earth from which it came. Just like you. Just like us all.

Triangle

"Geometry is not true, it is advantageous." – Herni
Poincare

There are an infinite number of triangles. While all geometric triangles share certain features, they all have 3 sides, 3 angles, and the sum of the 3 angles is precisely equal to 180 degrees. Otherwise the sides can be an infinite number of lengths which yield an infinite number of triangles. A similar statement can be made about the infinite number of triangle postures which could be practiced in yoga. While all triangle postures share some features, there are effectively an infinite number of ways that these features can be expressed. In other words, when you practice the triangle posture, your body does not have to look precisely like the triangle posture of other yoga practitioners or even teachers. Instead, practice finding both a feeling of grounding and stability coupled with a feeling of lift and lightness. Imagine the 3 farthest points of your body creating a triangle and then try changing the size of the angles and lines that connect them. For many people this will mean the heel of one foot (the back foot), the toes of the other foot (the front foot) and the fingertips of the topmost hand. For some people (who do not raise the top arm), the topmost point of the body may be the top shoulder or side of the head. This is where people sometimes get hung up on the idea of being able to "do the posture". Let go of this idea and instead just find the 3 farthest points. Then with each in breath expand the three points away from each other, or just lift the top most point. With each exhalation relax into the new found area of this expanded triangle (in geometry this is called a non-rigid transformation). The real point here is that the farthest

48

reaches of yourself and all the spaces in between are connected to each other. Their connection is illuminated when you practice yoga. If you are experiencing this connection then you are practicing triangle pose.

What other 3 pointed / 3 lined / 3 angled connections can you find in yourself. How about mind, breath, and body? What about left hip, right hip, and crown of your head? Left shoulder, right shoulder, and pelvic floor? Left fingertips, right finger tips, and crown of your head? Strengthen your awareness of their bonds and in so doing create an opportunity for strengthening the bonds themselves.

Hero

"I must not fear. Fear is the mind killer. It is the little death that brings total obliteration. I will face my fear. I will permit it to pass over me and through me. And when it has gone past, I will turn the inner eye to see its path. Where the fear has gone there will be nothing. Only I will remain."
– Frank Herbert

Heroic acts are not acts of confidence they are acts of courage. Heroism is the ability to act even in the face of seemingly unfavorable odds or even potential danger. Heroes are not super-humans who do not feel fear or uncertainty. Rather what makes them heroes is their ability to act in spite of a dearth of certainty and an abundance of fear. By the same token heroes are not out of touch with reality. Heroism is not blind action. Heroic acts are not engaged without regard for consequence. Again, the opposite is true. Heroic acts are undertaken knowing full well what the potential for success may be. Heroism is engaging with eyes open. Heroes are mindful and awake.

Ironically, when practicing the hero posture, there is no need to try to "be a hero". Instead move into the depth of your ankle and knee bend with mindfulness, fully aware of each sensation in those joints. Have the courage to slow down, to think through the best course of action and to evaluate possible outcomes. It is often the most courageous yoga practitioners who opt for the use of props to protect vulnerable parts of themselves from injurious actions. Protecting the weak is not weakness, it is strength. Forcing the weak to the whims of the strong is not strength, it is insecure bullying. Yes, you can act as a hero or a bully to the parts of yourself that need the most care and support.

Which will you choose to be? How will you know you've made this choice? The weakest parts of yourself, the places of uncertainty and fear will only learn to be strong if they are nurtured and cared for by your truest heroic self.

Staff

"What spectacle could be more edifying or more seasonable, than that of liberty and learning, each leaning on the other for their mutual and surest support?" – James Madison

Once again, let go of trying take the shape of this posture's namesake and instead embody the usefulness of this tool of human ingenuity. The staff is a tool of support. It aids in walking, in navigating uncertain terrain, and in rising from a seated to a standing position. The primary mechanism of these supports comes from the leveraged gained by driving the energy of the staff itself downward, creating an equal and opposite reaction of the body's motion upward. Create downward energy through your legs in the staff posture in order to facility the upward lift of your trunk. There is a steadiness to the staff. Create this feeling of steadiness as you gather the strength not only in your legs to press downward, but also in your abdomen to draw inward and your pelvic floor and muscles that run up the length of your spine to lift upward.

Gate

> "Still round the corner there may wait a new road or a
> secret gate, and though we may pass them by today,
> tomorrow we may come this way and take the hidden paths
> that run towards the Moon or the Sun." – J.R.R. Tolkien

Here in the gate posture we have yet another example of
how a yoga posture is not just one thing, or one position,
but has lots of room for variability and modulation. Every
gate is a break in a barrier, a way in or a way out. A gate
can be open or closed, locked or unlocked, entrance or exit,
a way to keep things in or let them out in a controlled way.
To be effective a gate must be mobile and fluid, but also
strong and stable.

Be strong and create stability as you bend and plant one leg
(either with toes tucked under or the top of your foot on the
ground, whichever is more stable for you) and lengthen and
plant the other leg stretched out the side. You will have
some room for adjustment with regard to the direction in
which the foot of the outstretched leg points, from facing
forward (the same direction in which your hips are facing)
all the way to facing straight outward to the side, and
anywhere in between. Choose the option for that foot that
allows you to feel stable with regard to your balance, but
also allows you to explore the freedom of movement in
your hip.

Mobilize the hip of your outturned leg. Stretch out along
the bent leg side of your body, including that arm as it
reaches out and overhead. Make room around your bottom
arm shoulder as you stretch out in its direction. Continue to
explore choices with regard to where you intentionally
open and where you deliberately close down. What are you

keeping in? What are you letting out? Do you need to open the gate a little wider to let something in or out? Do you need to keep the get shut and locked to keep something in or out? In any case, the choice is yours. You decide. You are the keeper of the gate.

Garland

"When you take a flower in your hand and really look at it,
it's your world for the moment." – Georgia O'Keefe

A garland is a collection of individual flowers strung
together into a unified whole. We cannot say with certainty
where the garland begins and ends. Likewise, each yoga
posture you practice is a collection of movements of
various parts of your body strung together into a unified
whole. Where does your body begin and end? What about
your mind? How about your breath? While each blossom in
the garland may be the same kind of flower, no two
blossoms are identical; each bloom is unique. In the same
way, while each inhalation or exhalation is quite similar to
all of the others, no two are identical; each breath is unique.
The same goes for thoughts and movements.

While you may repeat certain movements and postures
countless times, practicing them over and over again, no
two movements or performances of a posture will be
identical; each will be unique. While you bring consistency
to your practice you need not bring a rigid attitude about
performance.

As you practice the garland posture be like each individual
blossom and also be like the garland that brings them
together. Make mindful adjustments to the position of your
feet in the squatting position: as close together as all the
way touching, as wide apart as your hips, or anywhere in
between. Feel free to place support under your heels if they
do not touch the ground easily, or feel free to let them
hover. Be thoughtful with regard to the health of your
knees; do not strain them. Turn your feet to face the same
direction that your knees face. Feel free to sit upright or

bend forward between your legs. Place hands at your heart or stretch your arms out in front of you. Or, you might stretch arms in front of shins and out to the sides. You may even explore wrapping your arms around your legs and back behind you where fingers may or may not meet behind heels or across lower back. Whatever your garland looks like, it holds beauty. Enjoy it. Observe it. Meditate in it. Appreciate the garland and its many blossoms for what they are as individuals and a unified whole.

Dancer

"Think of the magic of that foot, comparatively small, upon which your whole weight rests. It's a miracle and the dance is a celebration of that miracle." – Martha Graham

Self expression through movement is the heart of dance. Dance is primarily expressive and creative and secondarily technical and precise. Furthermore, the practice of precision is only in the service of clearer and stronger expression.

Approach your practice of the dancer's posture from the inside out, rather than the outside in. Instead of trying to fit your body into an external model, create the model from the core of your being. Express your inner core of stability through your standing leg. Express the essence of your heart by lifting your chest to the sky. Like a dance duet, allow your arms and lifted leg to meet, forming a bond, a continuous cycle of give and take. There is a tension in dance that is contained and released repeatedly. Find this dynamic tension in your expression of the dancer's posture. Work with it. Mold it. Allow it to shape you.

Like a dancer moving to the rhythm of music, move your body with the rhythm of your breath and the music of your spirit. Listen intently while your breath keeps the beat steady and continuous. Dancers don't just hear the beat with their ears. A dancer listens with her/his whole body. In the same way, don't just listen to the sound of your breath flowing, feel the wave of its movement rising and falling within you and allow that cycle of motion to guide the actions of your body. In this way, dance and enjoy the dance.

Bow

"Happiness is a thing to be practiced, like the violin." –
John Lubbock

Sometimes people assume that yoga is all about relaxing, that tension has no place in a yoga practice. This view is missing an essential element of a practice of connecting and integrating. Tension is one way that connection is manifested. And particularly in the context of yoga, if that tension is intentional, then it is engaged in the service of connecting. There are numerous types of bows. What they have in common is more than in their names. Whether a bow associated with an arrow, or one used to play a violin, or even a string tied to hold shoes or presents together it is precisely the tension that gives the bow its power.

Instead of trying to eliminate all the tension in your being, practice harnessing the power of that tautness and utilizing it in the service of union. Use the tensile strength of your muscles to pull back, to push forward, and triangulate a center of balance. Just as you do not want to eliminate all opposing forces, you also do not want to only tighten. Like the archer stretching out the bow, relax into the pull. Like the virtuoso applying the pressure of the bow to the strings of the violin, relax into the beauty of the movement. Like the string tied to contain a gift, hold together, knowing that you have the intention to open and release.

Bridge

"Like a bridge over troubled water, I will lay me down." –
Simon and Garfunkle

The path your yoga practice takes is most likely not to be
linear. You can let go of the idea that you will continue to
make forward progress on your flexibility, your ability to
perform ever more challenging postures, and your
development of mental clarity and calm. Your practice will
sometimes feel like you have come to a dead stop. It is like
you have come to a seemingly insurmountable chasm. No
amount of brute force or ungrounded faith will allow you to
cross to the other side. Instead you will need to draw on
ingenuity and creativity to find a way across.

Even if you have not come to such a place in your practice,
you can prepare for this eventuality and be better equipped
to handle it by exploring the power of creative thought in
your practice of bridge. We tend to think of bridges only as
solid, stable structures when the bridges with the most
longevity are those that are both strong and have some
flexibility. Certainly embody the strength of a bridge as you
engage the power of your legs, upper back and shoulders.
But also find the mobility that allows your neck to find
ease, your heart to open, and your hips to lighten. Practice
being mentally flexible as well. Instead of thinking that you
must continue to push and struggle ever higher in your
hips, find instead that the beauty of the engineering is in the
kind of gentle bounce, the rise and fall that accompanies
your breath.

While you may be headed in a particular direction right
now, you know from experience that this direction will
inevitably change. Your path may even take you back along

the same route in the opposite direction. Instead of fighting this path, relax and embrace it. Bridges are made to connect across boundaries. The boundary crossing goes both ways. When you are traveling in one direction your point of view is focused in that direction. Even if you travel along the same route, but in the other direction you will experience that route in a whole new way. Likewise, while at first the energy of the bridge posture may be moving from feet to head, feel free to send the energy of movement back in the other direction. You will likely find a whole new experience of the bridge and of your own body.

Candle

"This little light of mine, I'm gonna let it shine." – Harry Dixon Loes

The purpose of a candle is to illuminate. The purpose of your yoga practice is to illuminate. The way that a candle works is that it slowly burns itself up in order to shed light. Better made candles burn slower and shed more light. Certainly you can practice building a better candle, with stronger shoulders, core, back, and legs, with freer shoulders, neck, chest and hip flexors. You could also build a better yoga practice, with increasing flexibility, strength, balance, range of motion, endurance, centeredness and focus. Yes, build a better candle. But then consider how you are using the light from that candle. Where will you choose to shine the light of your awareness? What do you see? How do you see it? Why do you see that and not something else? How do you use your light? Where do you choose to shine it? Why? How could you make better choices about how and where you shine your light? Yes, build a better yoga practice. But then consider how you are using the tool of your practice. The light of the candle does not just illuminate the candle. It is meant to light up the world around it. The light of your yoga practice does not only illuminate you. It is meant to light up the world around you.

Plow

"Those who profess to favor freedom and yet depreciate agitation are men who want crops without plowing up the ground." – Frederick Douglass

A plow simplifies digging. A plow makes it easier to plant seeds more plentifully and more successfully. A plow increases the probability of a higher yield of crops. But the primary purpose of a plow is to better ensure that those who benefit from its ultimate yield enjoy a greater bounty. Similarly in your practice of the plow posture you will likely find a stretch in your neck, shoulders, back, and hamstrings. You will probably enjoy building strength in your shoulders and core muscles. Whether you are aware of it or not, you will be promoting circulation by making it easier for veinous blood and lymph to return to your heart. In the upside down position you are strengthening your diaphragm, the muscle that facilities breathing. But the primary purpose of the plow posture is to better ensure that you will be able to enjoy a greater bounty of awareness. How deeply and widely you dig is up to you.

Wheel

"Unceasing change turns the wheel of life." - Amartya Sen

You don't have to look like a wheel to practice being a wheel. Where does a wheel begin? Where does a wheel end? Where does your practice of yoga begin? Where does it end? Choosing an entry point for your practice of yoga is like choosing an entry point for beginning movement around a wheel. It doesn't matter where you start. All that matters is that you enter, get the wheel of practice in motion and then continue to generate the energy necessary to keep the wheel spinning round and round.

Likewise, it doesn't really matter where your practice of the wheel posture begins. You can start with planting your feet firmly on the ground, or your hands near your shoulders, or breathing in and breathing out, or engaging the strength of your core muscles to stabilize your lower back, or expanding your heart, or focusing your mind in the present moment. Wherever you begin your practice of the wheel the other elements will follow in succession. So as not to battle yourself, decide on each particular round of practice in which direction the energy of the wheel will move; in other words, from your feet towards your hands, or from your hands towards your feet? Just like a spinning wheel, your body can move in either direction and once that direction is chosen, momentum will continue to drive the motion, so you'll likely want to avoid fighting against yourself.

As a reminder there is no way to "achieve/reach" the wheel pose. Instead there are only ways to practice embodying the circular energies of wheels. Let go of trying to reach a particular destination and embrace your engagement in the continuing journey that is yoga practice.

64

Acknowledgements

This book would not be possible without the long history of teachers and practitioners of yoga who have, with their bodies, with their very beings created this wondrous gift we call yoga. I am indebted to the Department of Social Sciences at the University of California, Irvine where I received my undergraduate degree in Political Science for NOT offering any coursework in public speaking. Without that oversight, I never would have taken the Speech For Drama course at UC Irvine where I first learned yoga. Although they didn't call what we practiced in that course "yoga" that is exactly what we were doing. Special thanks to those teachers in the drama department whose names I have forgotten, but whose impact upon my life and the lives of many others is indelible all the same.

I acknowledge Noll Daniel and Barbara Joseph for leading the first training course in yoga I took to become a "certified" yoga teacher at the Urban Yoga Center in New York City. My primary teachers have been the students who I have been honored to work with over the years. They have taught me honesty, kindness, compassion, caring, consideration, thoughtfulness, and how to be a more mindful human being.

This book would not be possible without the support of Jocelyn Dubin MS RD. She is my wife, best friend, and partner in life. She has encouraged me along my path as a teacher of yoga in countless ways and the writing of this book was no different. Jocelyn was also the primary editor of this book. Thank you Jocelyn.

And finally, thank you to the natural world and its many beings and thank you to the human beings whose creativity and compassion have benefited us all.

About The Author

Victor Dubin ERYT 500 has been a leader in yoga teaching since 1996 when he began a full time career teaching public yoga classes. He is co-founder of Nourish, a wellness center and yoga studio in Santa Cruz, California and has been a trainer of yoga teachers since 2001. His writing has been published in the book Yoga For Healthy Aging, by Baxter Bell MD and Nina Zolotow and on the Yoga For Healthy Aging and Yoga U Online blogs. In addition to teaching yoga, Victor is a stand-up comedian and has been a cross country coach, track and field coach, and a basketball coach. He lives with his wife and daughter in Santa Cruz, CA.